Cyber-Modeled-Health™ and Physiological Testing

John A. Allocca, D.Sc., Ph.D.

Published by
Allocca Biotechnology, LLC
www.allocca.com

updated: 12/22/14

Printed by www.createspace.com

ISBN 978-1-499-63958-2

Introduction

You do not need to understand everything in this training manual. The biochemical pathways are so complicated that a computer is required to analyze them.

What you need to understand is how to perform the testing. The software will do the rest.

Chapter 1 - Cyber-Modeled-Health™

Cyber-Modeled-Health™

"Cyber-Modeled-Health™" is a state-of-the-art scientific system that analyzes and addresses hundreds of biochemical pathways, biochemical models, and their interactions. Dr. Allocca developed this system in 1996 after 14 years of research and developing biochemical models. Most of the biochemical models used in the program are published in Dr. Allocca's textbook "Nutrition and Physiology with Biochemical Models."

Cyber-Modeled-Health™ also addresses the transport of nutrients from the blood into the cells, which may not happen automatically. People may be eating right and getting plenty of exercise, but if the critical process of transporting nutrients into the cells is not taking place, lactic acid can build up inside the cells damaging the cell membranes and DNA, which is the reason the body ages, organs degrade, and diseases begin.

The program produces an individualized step-by-step plan geared towards each persons needs to facilitate the appropriate changes for problems discovered including migraine, depression, bipolar disorder, carbohydrate craving, and more.

The approach to migraine and depression is twofold: remove the substances that are causing a loss of serotonin and norepinephrine and provide the brain with the raw ingredients it needs to make serotonin and norepinephrine.

The Cyber-Modeled-Health™ software is conveniently available online. After you complete the training course, you will get your own secure web page where you can process the data you collect and get a report in color instantly. You will also get a copy of each report in text format via email. This can be done from a PC, Mac, or other Portable device with an internet connection.

Parameters Analyzed

- Symptoms
- Height and Weight
- Zinc Taste Test
- Blood Pressure
- Daytime Core Temperature
- Urinalysis
- Bioelectric Impedance Analysis
- Peripheral Vascular Sonography
- Other Tests (optional)
- Microscopy (optional)

Cyber-Modeled-Health™ Report

- Client Information
- Conditions that may interfere with Good Health
- Zinc Sulfate Heptahydrate Test Results
- Calculated Basal Metabolic Rate
- Calculated Body Mass Index
- Daytime Core Temperature
- Urinalysis Results
- Bioelectric Impedance Analysis
- Symptoms Probability Profile
- Microscopy (if used)
- Other Tests (if used)
- Biometabolic Evaluation
- Food and Supplement Recommendations

Weight

Weight must be checked because most people lie about their weights.

Membrane Transport Mechanisms

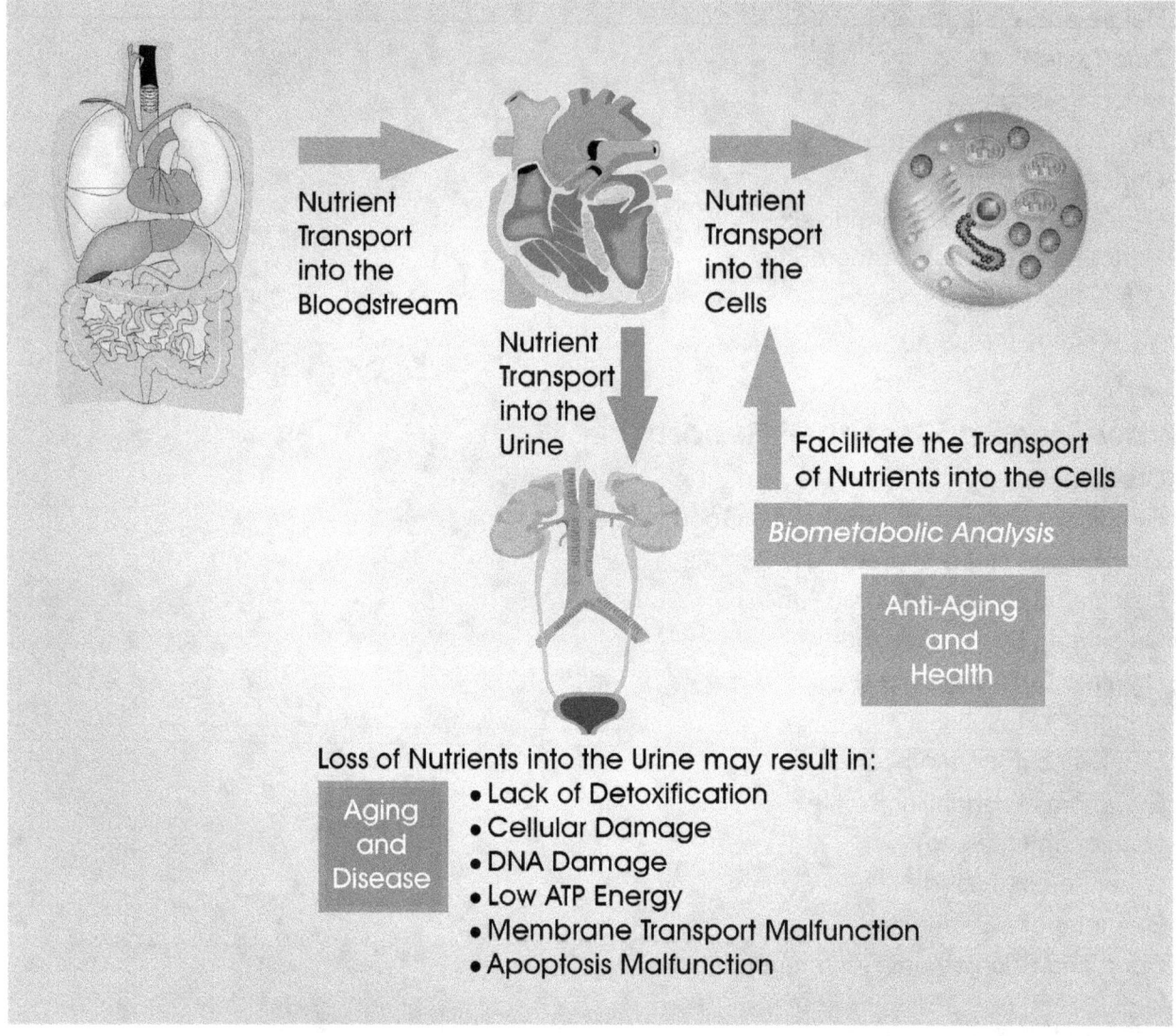

Nutrient Transport into the Bloodstream

Nutrient Transport into the Cells

Nutrient Transport into the Urine

Facilitate the Transport of Nutrients into the Cells

Biometabolic Analysis

Anti-Aging and Health

Loss of Nutrients into the Urine may result in:

Aging and Disease

- Lack of Detoxification
- Cellular Damage
- DNA Damage
- Low ATP Energy
- Membrane Transport Malfunction
- Apoptosis Malfunction

If all is working properly, nutrients are transported from the intestinal tract to the blood stream. Then, into the cells. Cyber-Modeled-Health™ facilitates this transport of nutrients into the cells.

If all is not working properly, nutrients are transported from the intestinal tract into the blood stream. Then, out of the body through the urinary system causing disease.

Detoxification Pathways

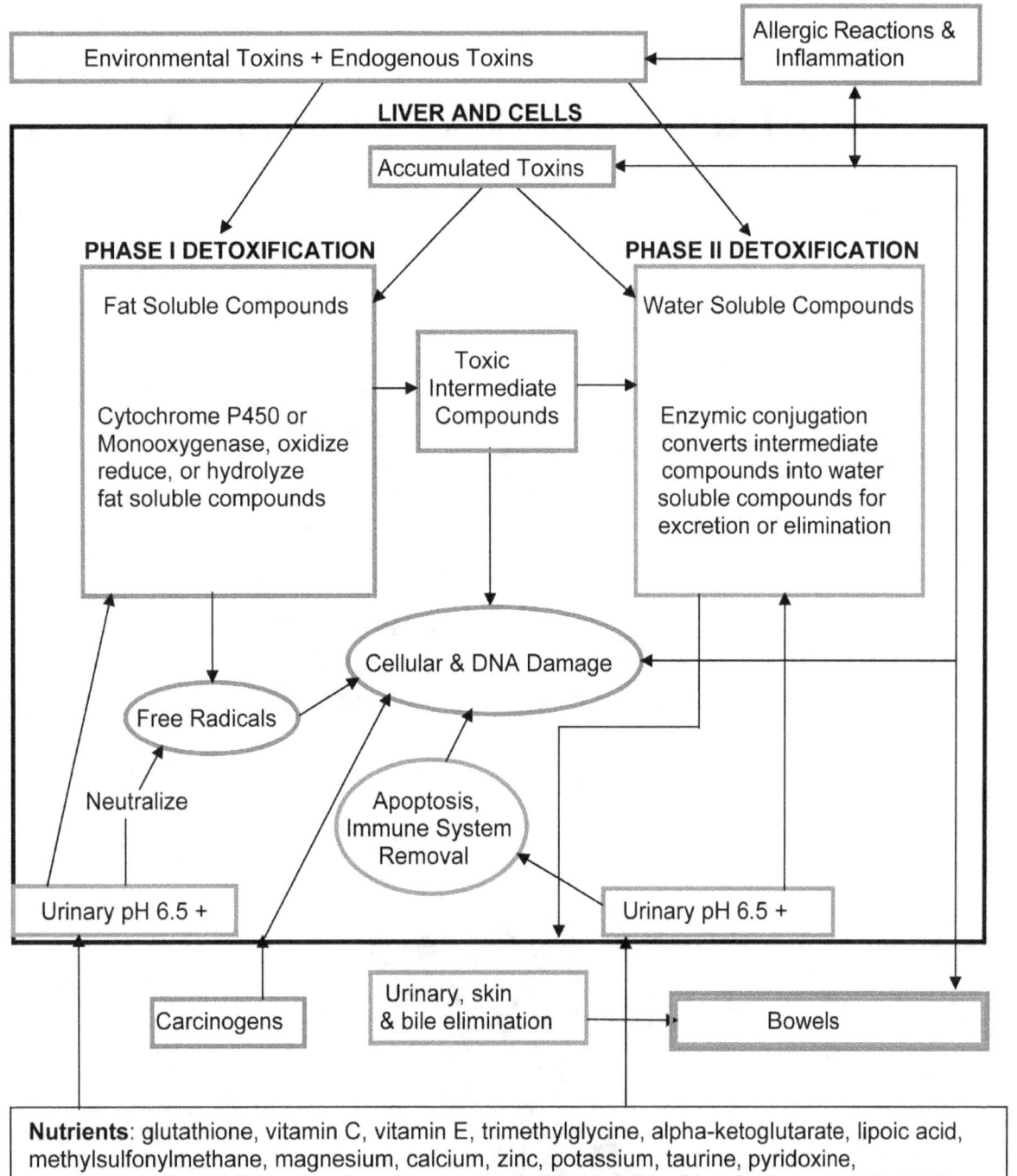

Above are some of the algorithms that are used in the program. Again, you do not need to understand this. It is so complicated that a computer is required to analyze all of the biochemical pathways.

Chapter 2 - Blood Pressure

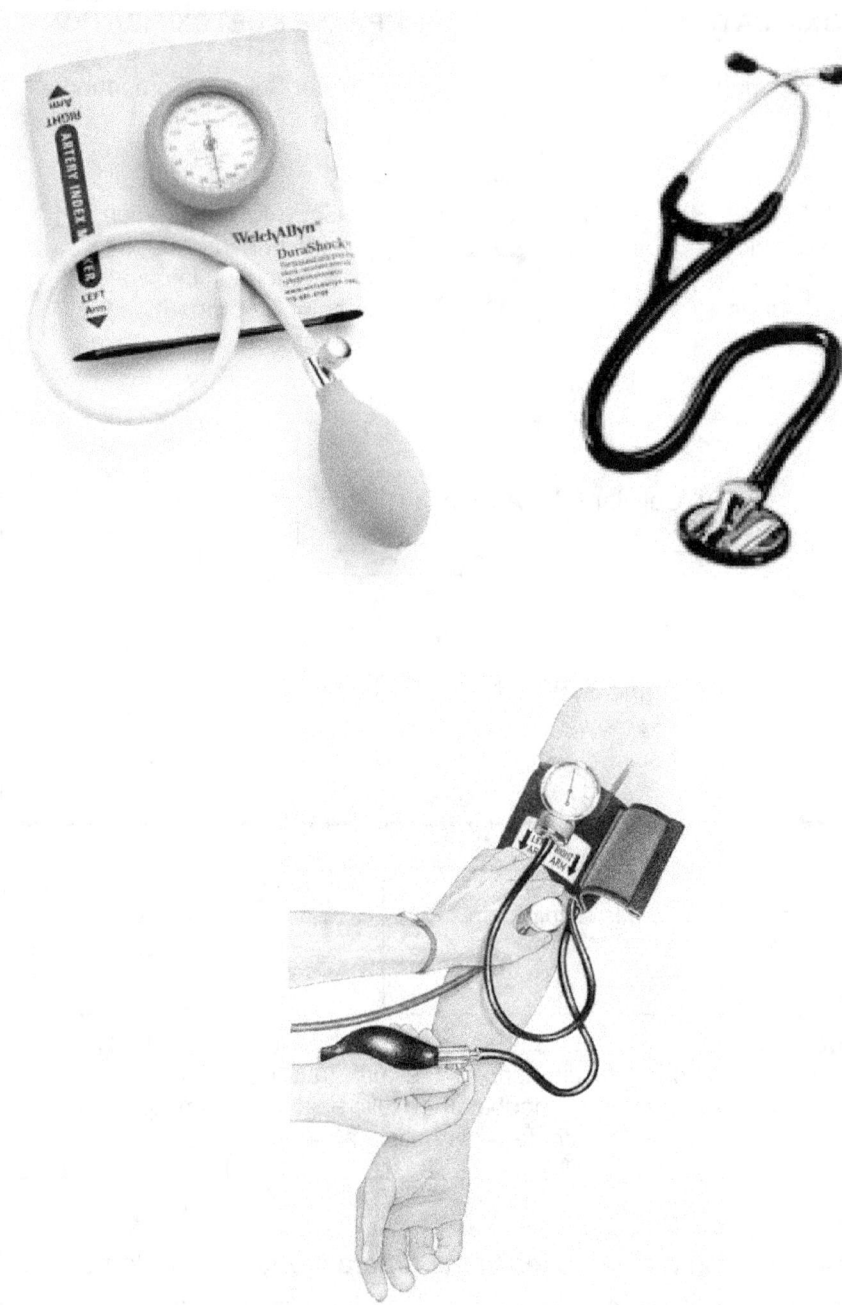

1. You will need a sphygmomanometer (blood pressure cuff, valve, and gage) of the appropriate size and stethoscope.

2. Apply the cuff around the patients arm approximately one inch above the elbow. Be sure to place the artery arrow inline with the brachial artery.

3. Place the stethoscope on the brachial artery at the anterior joint of the elbow. This is the point where the artery is closest to the surface. Place the other end of the stethoscope in your ears. Note that your ear canal is not straight into your head, but rather at angle towards the front. Your stethoscope should be made at this angle.

4. Tighten the valve on the sphygmomanometer.

5. Pump the bulb to inflate the cuff to about 150 mm Hg, while watching the dial.

6. Gently release the valve slightly to let the air out slowly.

7. Watch the dial and listen for the first heart beat. This is the systolic pressure. Remember it. If you do not hear a heart beat at 150 mm Hg, repeat the procedure and pump the cuff higher than 150 mm Hg.

8. Listen as the air releases for the point at which the sound disappears. The point just before the sound disappears is the diastolic pressure. Remember it.

9. Write down the two numbers as systolic/diastolic. For example, 120/70.

High blood pressure is considered as a pressure above 140/90.

Chapter 3 - Body Temperature

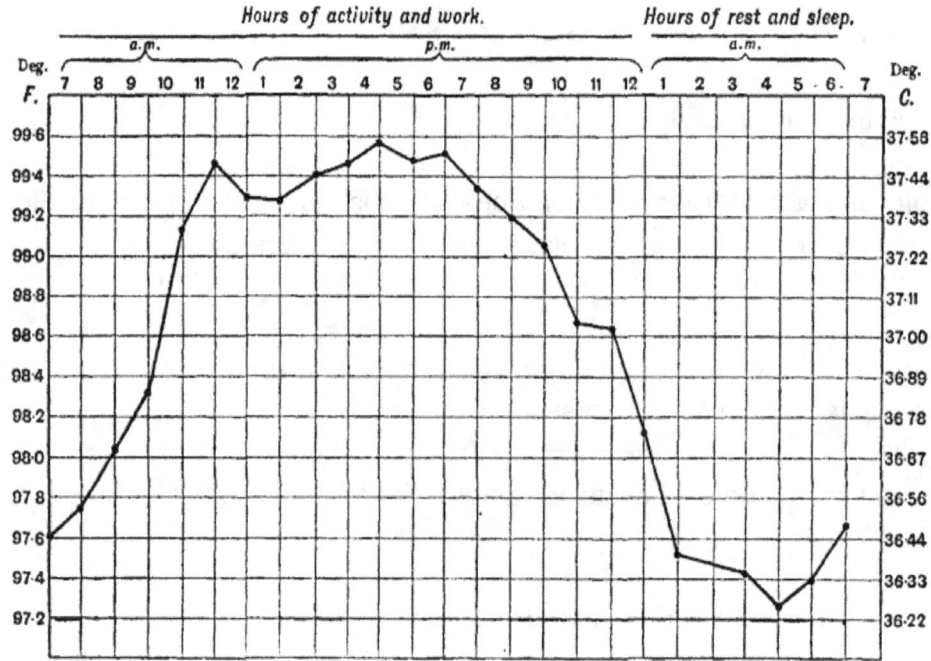

Core Body Temperature

Normal Daytime Temperature

Previously, average oral temperature for healthy adults had been considered 98.6° F, while the normal ranges is 97.0 to 100.0° F. Recent studies suggest that the average temperature for healthy adults is 98.2° F. Daily activity plays an important role in body temperature. The body temperature is the lowest during sleep and the highest during peak activity.

From 7 am to 1 am (chart above):
Normal Daytime Core Temperature (Ear):   97.8 to 99.6° F (36.6°-37.6° C)
Within 24 hours of ovulation, women experience an elevation of 0.2 - 0.9° F due to the increased metabolic rate caused by sharply elevated levels of progesterone. Women can chart this phenomenon to determine whether and when they are ovulating, so as to aid conception or contraception.

During strenuous exercise or extreme emotions, excessive body heat is produced. Body Temperature can temporarily rise as high as 101 to 104° F. When the body is exposed to extreme cold, the body temperature can fall to below 96° F.

The Braun ThermoScan Pro 4000 electronic ear thermometer is the instrument of choice for reliable measuring of core temperature. Studies have show the ear thermometer to be a reliable source for measuring core temperature.

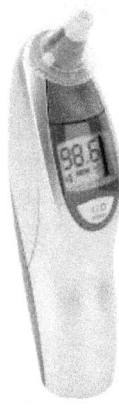

Basal Temperature Test for Thyroid Function

Basal (resting) body temperature is based on the work of Broda O. Barnes, M.D. during the 1970's Dr. Barnes correlated basal body temperature with basal metabolism on thousands of patients.

Basal (resting) Body Temperature is the temperature immediately upon awakening in the morning. Low basal temperature may be an indication of hypothyroidism. High basal temperature may be an indication of hyperthyroidism.

There are a number of methods for measuring basal temperature. The method that Dr. Barnes used was a mercury basal thermometer under the arm (axillary) for 10 minutes. By holding the thermometer under the arm for 10 minutes, Dr. Barnes brought the axillary temperature reading to become core temperature. Since that time, we have developed ear thermometers that are a quick and accurate means of measuring core temperature. According to the core temperature chart above, temperature at rest and sleep should begin at 97.8° F, which is identical to Dr. Barnes's figure of 97.8° F.

Normal Basal Axillary temperature (Dr. Barnes) = 97.8° F to 98.2° F (36.6° C to 36.8° C)

A basal temperature below 97.8° F (36.6° C) strongly suggests under-active thyroid function.

A basal temperature above 98.2° F (36.8° C) strongly suggests an infection or overactive thyroid function.

For men, average 5 days. For women, average days 2 and 3 or their menstrual cycle.

Women should mark the 1st, 2nd and 3rd day of their menstrual cycle on the chart. In women, temperature changes as the levels of reproductive hormones change. Temperatures rise between 0.4 and 0.8° F on the day of ovulation. During the luteal phase (post ovulatory phase) of the cycle, the corpus luteum produces the hormone progesterone, which elevates the basal temperature. When the basal temperature has gone up for several days, ovulation has occurred. The basal temperature for thyroid and adrenal function evaluation is an average of the 2nd and 3rd day.

Do not take a temperature reading within 36 hours of taking aspirin, ibuprofen, Tylenol, or similar antipyretic. There are a number of drugs and nutritional supplements that lower body temperature. If there is a significant variation in temperature, use the peak readings.

Reference

"Hypothyroidism: The Unsuspected Illness," Broda O. Barnes, M.D. and Lawrence Galton, Harer & Row Publishers, New York, 1976.

Basal Temperature Chart

Name:_____

Measure temperature upon awakening. 5 days for men, 30 days for women.
If you are sleeping with substantial covers, your temperature should be taken 10 minutes or so after uncovering. Do not take a temperature reading within 36 hours of taking aspirin, ibuprofen, Tylenol, or similar antipyretic. There are a number of drugs and nutritional supplements that lower body temperature. If there is a significant variation in temperature, use the peak readings.

Date	Temp.	Date	Temp.	Date	Temp.
_____	_____	_____	_____	_____	_____
_____	_____	_____	_____	_____	_____
_____	_____	_____	_____	_____	_____
_____	_____	_____	_____	_____	_____
_____	_____	_____	_____	_____	_____
_____	_____	_____	_____	_____	_____
_____	_____	_____	_____	_____	_____
_____	_____	_____	_____	_____	_____
_____	_____	_____	_____	_____	_____
_____	_____	_____	_____	_____	_____
_____	_____	_____	_____	_____	_____
_____	_____	_____	_____	_____	_____

Chapter 4 - Zinc Sulfate Heptahydrate Test

The zinc taste test uses a non-toxic zinc solution of zinc sulfate in purified water, at a concentration of 1gm/liter.

The solution should be stored in a refrigerator and discarded after six months.

The solution should be removed from storage and left at room temperature for about two hours before the test.

Test

No food or drink 1 hour before the test.

1. Pour about 10 ml (2 teaspoons) of solution into a cup.

2. Have the patient place it in his/her mouth and swish it around for about 10 seconds. Then swallow.

3. Ask the patient if her/she has experienced a sour or metallic taste.

Results

No specific taste sensation: tastes like plain water. This indicates a low level of zinc in the body.

A metallic or sour taste indicates an adequate level of zinc in the body.

Chapter 5 - Urinalysis

A Fresh sample should be used.
No food 4 hours before test.
No alcohol 24 hours before test.

Appearance

Normal urine is clear. Cloudy urine indicates infectious solutes (WBC's, pus, bacteria) or it is too alkaline.

Color

Colorless indicates a high water intake or anemia or bile deficiency.
Yellow is normal.

Dark Yellow indicates dehydration or antibiotic use or Vitamins A, B supplements or fasting and has high fever.

Yellow-brown or Yellow-green indicates bile pigments in urine or from drugs.

Red or Red-brown caused by eating beets or hemoglobin in the urine or from some medications.

Orange-red or Orange-brown indicates presence of urobilinogen in the urine or from drugs.

Dark-brown or Black indicates malanins or dark pigments of tumors in the urinary tract or the presence of iron portion of hemoglobin in the urine.

Specific Gravity (1.016 - 1.022)

Osmolality (concentration). above 1.022 indicates renal dysfunction or dehydration.

pH (5 - 7)

Above 7 indicates metabolic alkalosis or infection or diet high in alkaline ash.
Below 5 indicates metabolic acidosis or high stress or excessive stimulants (Caffeine, alcohol, drugs).

Leukocytes (0)

Positive indicates infection or high Vitamin C intake.

Nitrite (0)

Bacteria convert nitrate to nitrite in the urine. Presence of nitrite indicates bacterial infection of the kidney or urinary tract.

Protein (0 - 30 mg/dl)

Above 30 mg/dl indicates renal dysfunction or excessive protein in the diet or strenuous exercise or emotional stress or during fever or exposure to excessive heat or cold. Protein in the urine for a prolonged period of time indicates renal dysfunction.

Glucose (0)

The kidney's will reabsorb all the glucose in the urine as long as the level is below 160 - 190 mg %. Positive glucose in the urine indicates diabetes.

Ketones (0)

When glucose is not available during fasting, adipose tissue triglycerides are reconverted to free fatty acids and glycerol (lipolysis). When the fatty acids are metabolized, ketone bodies are produced as an energy source for the brain and other tissues when glucose is not available. Positive indicates fasting or carbohydrate starvation or vomiting or diarrhea or diabetes or excessive alcohol use.

Urobilinogen (less than 1 mg/dl)

Bacteria in the intestinal tract reduce bilirubin to urobilinogen. Urobilinogen is present in the urine in trace amounts. Antibiotics and drugs destroy the intestinal flora and cause an absence of urobilinogen in the urine and feces. It is also absent in obstructive jaundice where no bilirubin reaches the intestinal tract to be converted to urobilinogen.

    Increased blood cell destruction increases bilirubin and the subsequent conversion to urobilinogen.

    Above 1 indicates hemolytic anemia or pernicious anemia or sickle cell anemia

    Absence indicates reduced intestinal flora or liver dysfunction or biliary obstruction.

Bilirubin (0 - 0.5 mg/dl)

Bilirubin is formed as result of the breakdown of damaged or worn out red blood cells in the spleen and bone marrow. After hemoglobin is released, it is converted into globin and heme. Heme is converted to bilirubin after the iron is removed for recycling. After passing through the liver, the protein-bound bilirubin is made water soluble and passes into the intestines through the bile duct where it emulsifies fats. When found in the urine, it indicates excess bilirubin in the blood.

    Positive indicates liver dysfunction or biliary obstruction.

Blood (0 - 5 Erythrocytes/ul)

There should not be any red blood cells (erythrocytes) in the urine.
Positive indicates menstruation or infection or strenuous exercise or exposure to excessive cold or renal dysfunction or drugs. Follow up with microscopic exam.

Note: The above analysis is available on a single reagent test strip.

Indican

Indican is formed by an abnormal metabolism of tryptophan. Indican is a by-product of putrefaction (protein degradation), usually in the intestine. Putrefaction is the anaerobic bacterial decomposition of proteins.

When the product of this putrefaction (indole) is absorbed into the blood stream, an increase in urinary indican is seen. This increase can also be seen if bacterial decomposition of body tissues or fluids occurs, as in gangrene, abscesses, etc.

Among the pathologic conditions in which urinary indican is likely to be elevated are hypochlorhydria (low stomach acid production), inhibited peristaltic movement (the involuntary muscular "waves" that move food through your bowel), and poor production of digestive bile secretions from the gall bladder and liver. Elevated indican is rather rare in simple constipation, but often high with diarrhea. It is generally a good indicator for the poor breakdown of proteins accompanied by increased intestinal permeability (leaky gut).

Bayer Multistix 10 SG Reagent Strip Urinalysis

Manufacturer's Number 2161

Use a Fresh Urine Sample Only

Name_____

Date_____

INSTRUCTIONS

1. Dip reagent strip into a fresh urine sample.

2. Wait two minutes.

3. Circle the Matching Colors

4. Discard the test strip

Place Your Strip Here

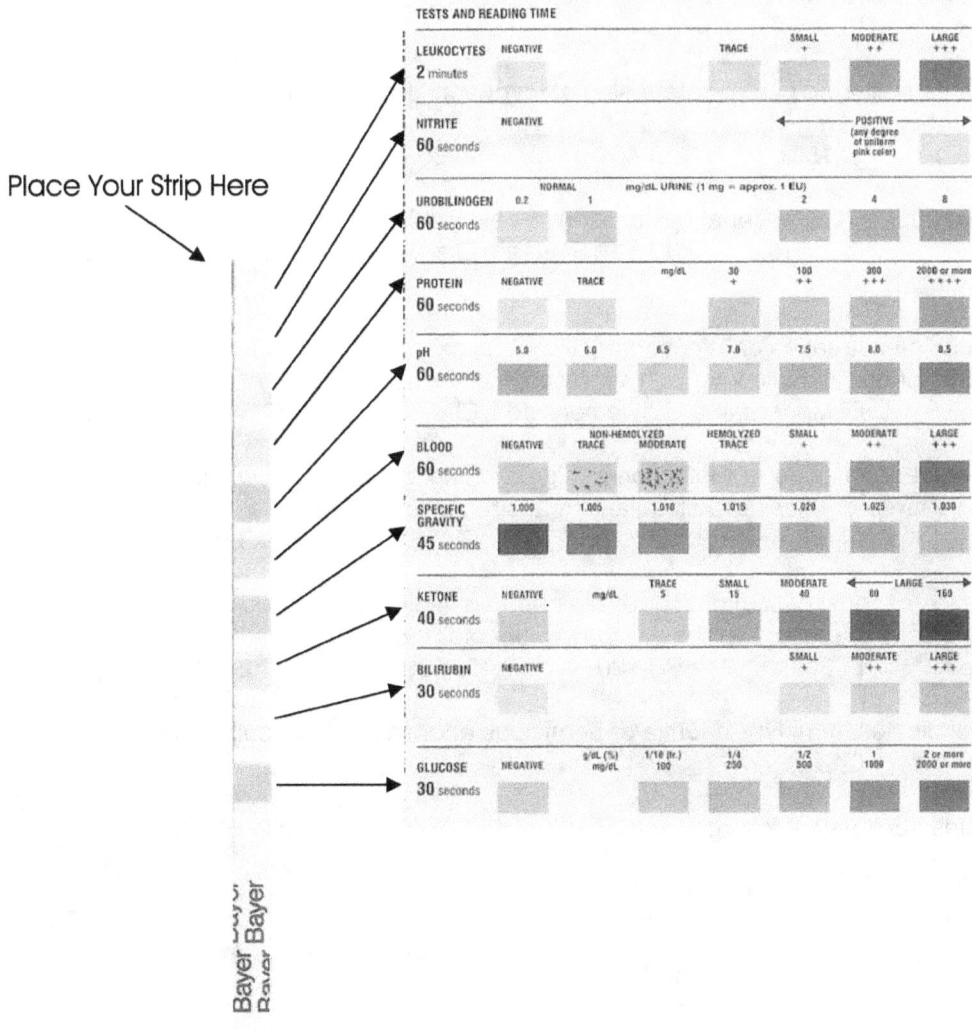

Urinalysis - Fresh Collection

Client's Name:_____

Appearance:
☐ Cloudy (Infection or too alkaline)
☐ Clear (Normal)

Color:
☐ Colorless (High water intake or anemia or bile deficiency)
☐ Yellow (Normal)
☐ Dark Yellow (Dehydration or antibiotics or Vitamin A, B supplements or fasting & high fever)
☐ Yellow-brown or Yellow-green (Bile pigments present or drugs)
☐ Red or Red-brown (Eating beets or hemoglobin present or medications)
☐ Orange-red or Orange-brown (Urobilinogen present or drugs)
☐ Dark-brown or Black (Malanins or tumors or iron/hemoglobin present)

Glucose (Positive indicates diabetes) mg/dl
☐ Negative   ☐ 100   ☐ 250   ☐ 500   ☐ 1000   ☐ 2000 or more

Bilirubin (Positive indicates liver dysfunction or biliary obstruction)
☐ Negative   ☐ +   ☐ ++   ☐ +++

Ketones (Positive indicates fasting or carbohydrate starvation or vomiting or diabetes or diarrhea or diabetes or excessive alcohol use) mg/dl
☐ Negative   ☐ 5   ☐ 15   ☐ 40   ☐ 80   ☐ 160

Specific Gravity (Above 1.022 indicates renal dysfunction or dehydration)
☐ 1.000   ☐ 1.005   ☐ 1.010   ☐ 1.015   ☐ 1.020   ☐ 1.025   ☐ 1.030

Blood (Positive indicates menstruation or infection or strenuous exercise or renal dysfunction or exposure to excessive cold or drugs. Follow up with microscopic exam)
☐ Negative   ☐ Trace   ☐ Moderate   ☐ Hemolyzed   ☐ +   ☐ ++   ☐ +++

pH (Above 7 indicates metabolic alkalosis or infection or high alkaline ash diet. Below 5 indicates metabolic acidosis or high stress or excessive stimulants (caffeine, alcohol, drugs)
☐ 5.0   ☐ 6.0   ☐ 6.5   ☐ 7.0   ☐ 7.5   ☐ 8.0   ☐ 8.5

Protein (Above trace indicates renal dysfunction or excess protein in diet or strenuous exercise or emotional stress or high fever or exposure excessive to heat or cold) mg/dl
☐ Negative   ☐ Trace   ☐ 30   ☐ 100   ☐ 300   ☐ 2000 or more

Urobilinogen (Above 1 indicates hemolytic anemia or pernicious anemia or sickle cell anemia) mg/dl
☐ 0.2   ☐ 1   ☐ 2   ☐ 4   ☐ 8

Nitrite (Positive indicates bacterial infection)
☐ Negative   ☐ Positive

Leukocytes (Positive indicates infection or high Vitamin C intake)
☐ Negative   ☐ Trace   ☐ +   ☐ ++   ☐ +++

Reference: *Bayer* Multistix 10 SG urine reagent strips

Chapter 6 - Bioelectrical Impedance Analysis (BIA)

A small alternating current (usually 50 KHz.) is passed through the body via attached electrodes. Resistance and reactance are measured to obtain tissue conductivity, phase angles, etc.

Patient Pre-Test Instructions

1. No alcohol consumption within 24 hours prior to the test.

2. No exercise, caffeine, or food within 4 hours prior to the test.

3. Drink 2 glasses of water 2 hours before the test.

BIA Measurement Procedure

1. Switch the unit on and allow it to calibrate.

2. Enter "Guest"

3. Enter the patient's age, set. Sex, set, and height, but don't press set yet.

4. Have the patent step onto the measurement platform and have them place their feet on the foot electrodes with weight evenly distributed. Haven them raise their arms. Then, press set.

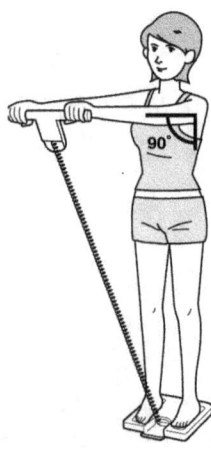

5. The display will show the weight and then the weight result will blink twice. Then, The monitor will start to calculate body composition.

6. When the measurement is completed, the weight is displayed again. Step off the measurement platform.

Body Mass Index (Weight)

Body Mass Index is equal to the ratio of the body's weight in kilograms to the square of height in meters. A BMI over 25 indicates that the individual is overweight. The obesity guideline from the National Heart, Lung, and Blood Institute of the National Institutes of Health proposes that practitioners use body mass index (BMI) to assess patients because the index is simple, correlates to fatness, and applies to both men and women.

Body Mass Index = Weight in kilograms / (Height in meters)^2

Body Mass Index = (Weight in pounds / 2.2) / (Height in inches / 39.37)^2

Ideal Weight = (BMI x (Height in inches / 39.37)^2) x 2.2

The National Heart, Lung, and Blood Institute proposes the following classifications of health using body mass index:

Body Mass Index	Classification
Less than 18.5	Underweight
18.5 to 24.9	Normal
25.0 to 29.9	Overweight
30.0 to 34.9	Obese Class I
35.0 to 39.9	Obese Class II
40.0 or greater	Extremely Obese

Mass Distribution (Body Composition)

Mass Distribution - The body as a whole is made up of fat-free mass and fat mass.

Body Fat Mass

Fat Mass (Body Fat) is the total amount of stored lipids in the body and consists of subcutaneous fat and visceral fat. Subcutaneous Fat is located directly beneath the skin and serves as an energy reserve and as insulation against outside cold. Visceral Fat is located deeper within the body and serves as an energy reserve and as a cushion between organs. High body fat can lead to cardiovascular and other disorders.

Body fat serves a vital role in storing energy and protecting internal organs. We carry two types of fat in our bodies: 1) essential fat which is stored in small amounts to protect the body and 2) stored fat which is stocked for energy during physical activity. While too much body fat may be unhealthy, having too little fat can be just as unhealthy. low body fat may have dry skin, increased cold sensitivity, reduced energy, hair loss, impaired immune system function and increased bruising. Also, the distribution of body fat in men and women is different, so the basis for classifying the body fat percentage is different between the genders. Source: NIH/WHO guidelines for BMI.

Source: Gallagher et al., American Journal of Clinical Nutrition, Vol. 72, Sept. 2000.

Interpreting the Body Fat Percentage Result

Gender	Age	Low (–)	Normal (0)	High (+)	Very High (++)
Female	20-39	< 21.0	21.0 - 32.9	33.0 - 38.9	≥ 39.0
	40-59	< 23.0	23.0 - 33.9	34.0 - 39.9	≥ 40.0
	60-79	< 24.0	24.0 - 35.9	36.0 - 41.9	≥ 42.0
Male	20-39	< 8.0	8.0 - 19.9	20.0 - 24.9	≥ 25.0
	40-59	< 11.0	11.0 - 21.9	22.0 - 27.9	≥ 28.0
	60-79	< 13.0	13.0 - 24.9	25.0 - 29.9	≥ 30.0

Skeletal Muscle Mass

Skeletal muscle is the type of muscle that we can see and feel. When you work out to increase muscle mass, skeletal muscle is being exercised. Skeletal muscles attach to the skeleton and come in pairs -- one muscle to move the bone in one direction and another to move it back the other way. Increasing skeletal muscle will increase your body's energy requirements. The more muscle you have, the more calories your body will burn. Building skeletal muscle can help prevent "rebound" weight gain. The maintenance and increase of skeletal muscle is closely linked to resting metabolism rate.

Interpreting the Skeletal Muscle Percentage Result

Gender	Age	Low (−)	Normal (0)	High (+)	Very High (++)
Female	18-39	< 24.3	24.3 - 30.3	30.4 - 35.3	≥ 35.4
	40-59	< 24.1	24.1 - 30.1	30.2 - 35.1	≥ 35.2
	60-80	< 23.9	23.9 - 29.9	30.0 - 34.9	≥ 35.0
Male	18-39	< 33.3	33.3 - 39.3	39.4 - 44.0	≥ 44.1
	40-59	< 33.1	33.1 - 39.1	39.2 - 43.8	≥ 43.9
	60-80	< 32.9	32.9 - 38.9	39.0 - 43.6	≥ 43.7

Visceral Fat Mass

Visceral Fat is found in the abdomen and surrounding vital organs. It is different from fat found directly underneath the skin, which is referred to as subcutaneous fat. Visceral fat can go largely unnoticed because it's not visible to the naked eye. Too much visceral fat is thought to be closely linked to increased levels of fat in the bloodstream, which may lead to conditions such as high cholesterol, heart disease and type 2 diabetes. In order to prevent or improve these conditions, it is important to try to reduce the amount of visceral fat levels to an acceptable level.

Interpreting the Visceral Fat Level Result

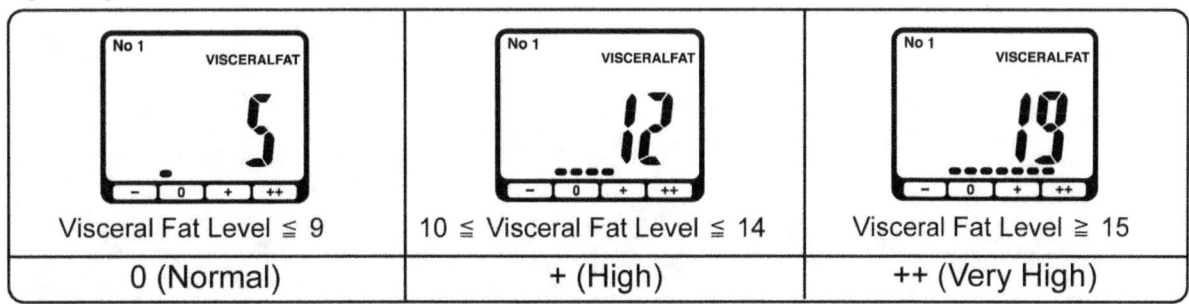

Visceral Fat Level ≤ 9	10 ≤ Visceral Fat Level ≤ 14	Visceral Fat Level ≥ 15
0 (Normal)	+ (High)	++ (Very High)

Basal Metabolic Rate

Basal Metabolic Rate is the rate the body burns energy (calories) during a normal resting state, over a 24-hour period. Basal metabolic rate is the key to effective weight management. Basal Metabolic Rate indicates more than 90% of total daily energy expenditure. Bioelectric Impedance Analyzers determine the basal metabolic rate by fat-free mass since only fat-free mass is metabolized.

BMR (calories/day) = 14.15 x Fat-Free Mass (pounds)

BMR (calories/day) = 31.2 x Fat-Free Mass (kilograms)

Caloric expenditure is elevated during exercise and occupational activity, which provides the benefit of maintaining fat-free mass.

Instrument Recommendation

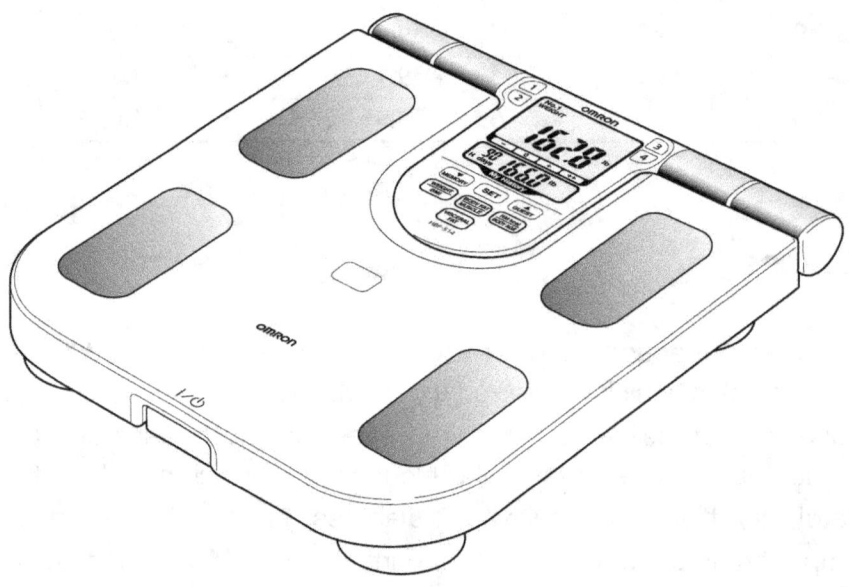

Omron HBF-514C

Chapter 7 - Blood Glucose

Glucose is the form of carbohydrate that is used by the tissue and brain cells. Insulin transports excess glucose from the blood into cells. A high level primarily indicates diabetes mellitus or pancreatitis. A low level primarily indicates hyperinsulinism, functional hypoglycemia, protein malnutrition, medications, sometimes in alcoholism. The normal range is 70-100 mg/dl based on a 4 hour fast.

Measurement Procedure

1. Insert the lancet into the lancing device and remove the protective cover.

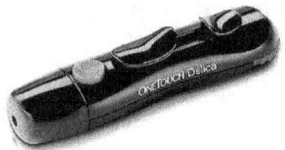

2. Insert the test strip into the glucose meter (glucometer) - Freestyle Lite Glucose meter.

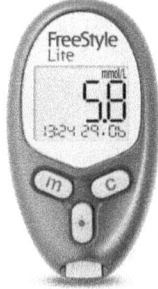

3. Wipe the patient's finger with an alcohol prep.

4. Place the lancing device on the side of the finger. Then, press the button.

5. Apple the finger with blood to the test strip. Record the reading.

Chapter 8 - Peripheral Vascular Sonography

Reducing the risk factors that lead to peripheral artery disease is critical to stop progression, such as reducing cholesterol and blood pressure, not smoking, and eating a healthy low fat diet. Aspirin may be prescribed or other anticlotting drugs. The most effective treatment is exercise. In cases of severe peripheral artery disease, surgery can bypass a blocked artery and restore blood flow. Peripheral artery disease is dangerous, even when it's silent. Even when symptoms are not noticeable, people with peripheral artery disease decrease their activity level over time. Peripheral artery disease is proof that atherosclerosis is occurring throughout the body. Even if peripheral artery disease never causes problems itself, it increases the risk of dying from heart attack or stroke significantly.

Doppler ultrasound devices are used to measure the blood flowing in peripheral arteries. Peripheral artery disease (PAD) occurs when the blood vessels become narrow from the build up of plaque along the artery walls, which is referred to as atherosclerosis. PAD most commonly occurs in the legs, feet, and toes.

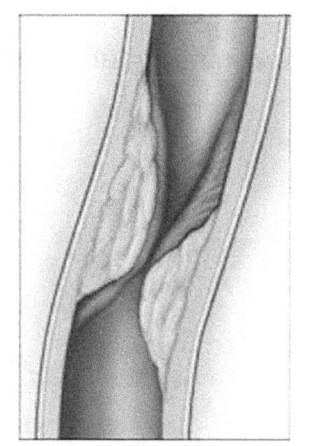

Artery narrowed by plaque

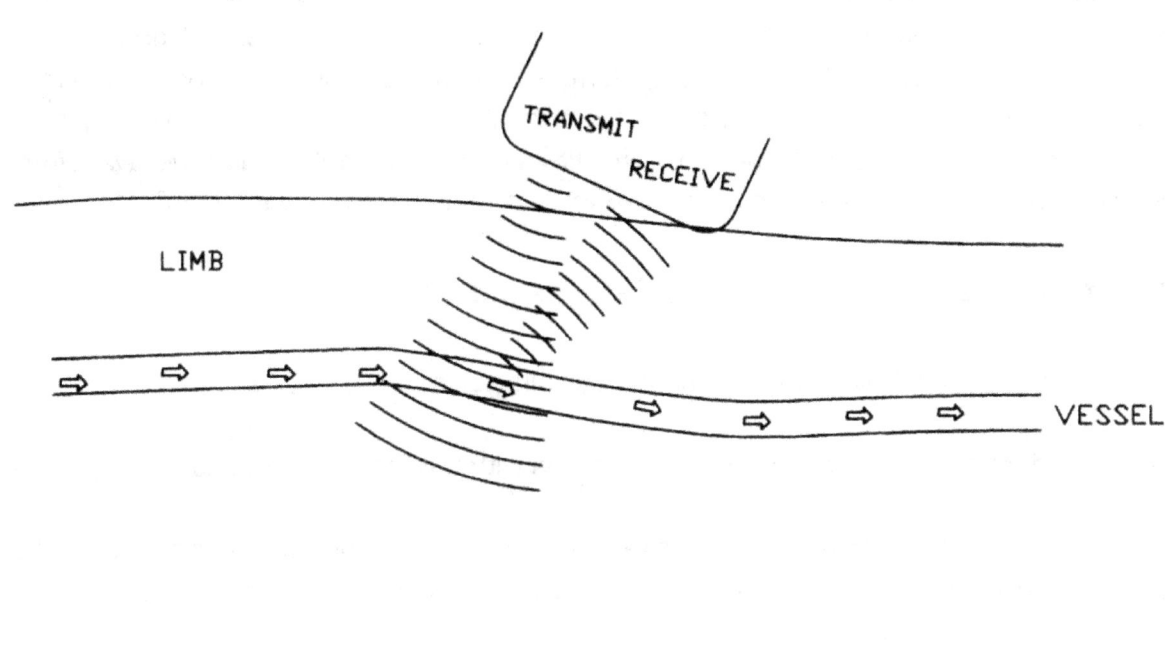

LIMB

TRANSMIT

RECEIVE

VESSEL

Waveform Analysis

The ultrasonic or doppler waveform follows the blood flow pulse of arteries. The analyses ultrasonic or doppler waveforms provide information for assessing the extent and location of peripheral vascular disease. The normal waveform is triphasic and includes forward and reverse (diastolic) components. With progression of disease, the reverse component is lost, and the waveform becomes biphasic. When forward flow becomes continuous, the waveform is considered monophasic. In severe disease, the waveform amplitude is dampened.

Characteristics of a normal arterial waveform

1. A sharp rise in the upstroke representing the systolic pulse.

2. A more gradual decline during diastole, sometimes with bowing during diastole.

3. A dicrotic notch in the diastolic down stroke in waveforms of blood vessels close to the heart, such as the carotid and brachial arteries will show the dichotic notch (the closing of the aortic valve) in a healthy individual.

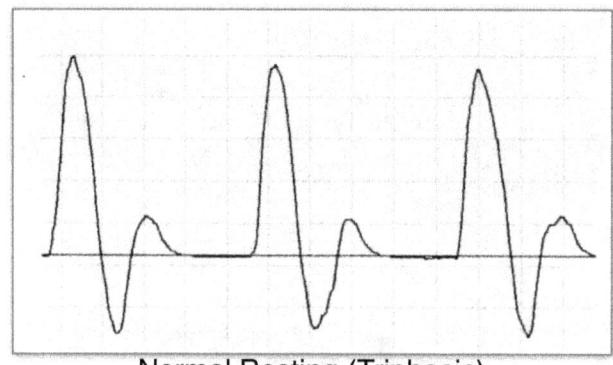

Normal Resting (Triphasic)

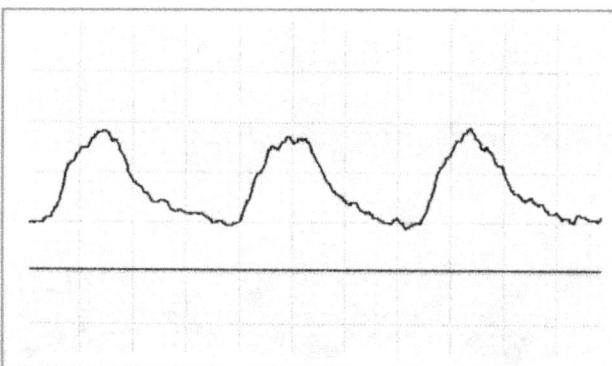

Early diastolic flow reversal (Biphasic)

Prolonged systolic upstroke, pandiastolic forward flow without diastolic flow reversal (monophasic)

30

Measure the Brachial Artery Waveform and Pressure

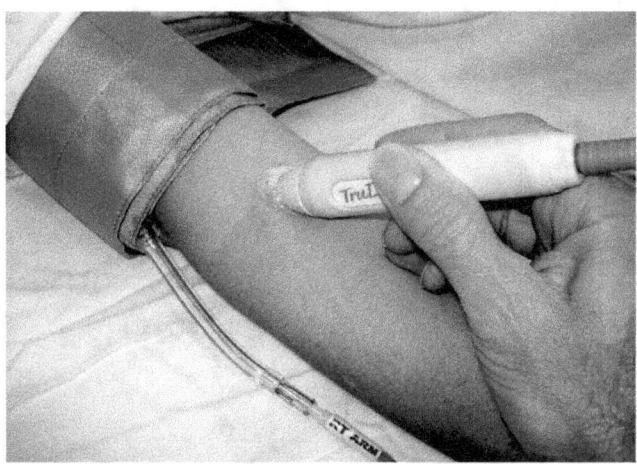

1. Have the patient rest horizontally for 5 minutes.

2. Place 12 cm blood pressure cuffs on the arms and the 10 cm cuffs on the ankles. Do not inflate the cuffs at this time.

3. Place ultrasound gel on the skin above the left brachial artery as shown above.

4. Gently place the Doppler probe over the left brachial artery. Do not apply pressure. Hold the probe above the artery at a 45 to 60 degree angle against flow. Adjust the probe angle until the best sound is heard and a steady waveform appears on the LCD.

5. Record the type of waveform on the ABI Form (Triphasic, Biphasic, Monophasic, Diminished Monophasic).

6. Print the waveform if abnormal.

7. Take the systolic pressure by inflating the cuff to 20 mmHg over pressure (sound) cessation. Then, slowly deflate the cuff at a rate of 2-3 mmHg per second until the first Doppler sound is heard and waveform motion on the LCD returns.

8. Record the pressure on the ABI Form.

9. Repeat steps 3 through 8 for the right brachial artery.

Note: It doesn't matter if you start on the left of the right.

Measure the Posterior Tibial Artery Waveform and Pressure

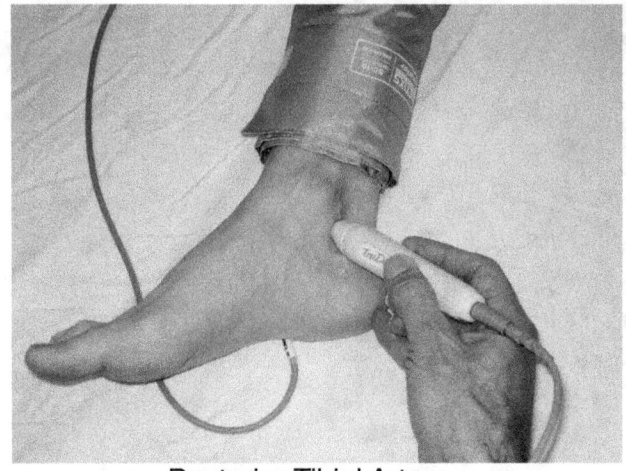 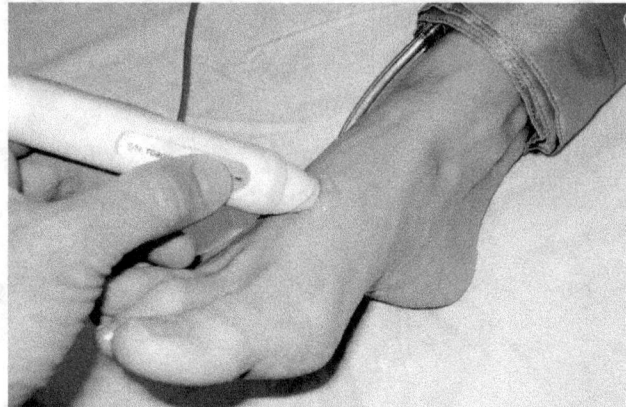

Posterior Tibial Artery   Dorsalis Pedis Artery

1. Apply ultrasound gel to the skin above the left posterior tibial artery as shown above.

2. Gently place the Doppler probe over the left posterior tibial artery. Do not apply pressure. Hold the probe above the artery at a 45 to 60 degree angle against flow. Adjust the probe angle until the best sound is heard and a steady waveform appears on the LCD. If waveform cannot be obtained from the left posterior tibial, use the left dorsalis pedis artery.

3. Record the type of waveform on the ABI Form (Triphasic, Biphasic, Monophasic, Diminished Monophasic).

4. Print the waveform.

5. Take the systolic pressure by inflating the cuff to 20 mmHg over pressure (sound) cessation. Then, slowly deflate the cuff at a rate of 2-3 mmHg per second until the first Doppler sound is heard and waveform motion on the LCD returns.

6. Record the pressure on the ABI Form.

7. Repeat steps 1 trough 6 for the right posterior tibial artery.

Note: It doesn't matter if you start on the left of the right.

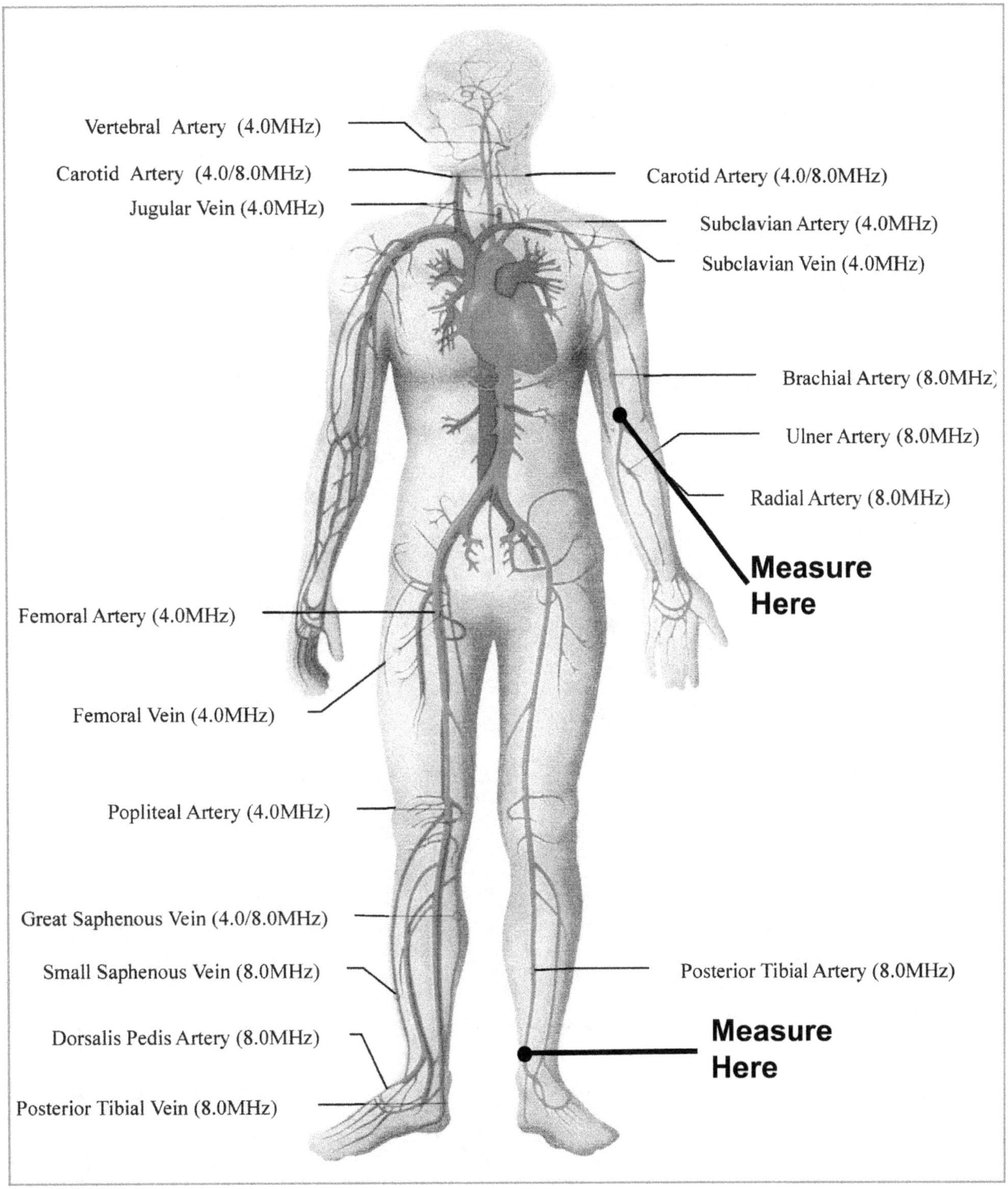

Vertebral Artery (4.0MHz)

Carotid Artery (4.0/8.0MHz)

Jugular Vein (4.0MHz)

Carotid Artery (4.0/8.0MHz)

Subclavian Artery (4.0MHz)

Subclavian Vein (4.0MHz)

Brachial Artery (8.0MHz)

Ulner Artery (8.0MHz)

Radial Artery (8.0MHz)

**Measure
Here**

Femoral Artery (4.0MHz)

Femoral Vein (4.0MHz)

Popliteal Artery (4.0MHz)

Great Saphenous Vein (4.0/8.0MHz)

Small Saphenous Vein (8.0MHz)

Dorsalis Pedis Artery (8.0MHz)

Posterior Tibial Vein (8.0MHz)

Posterior Tibial Artery (8.0MHz)

**Measure
Here**

Calculate ABI

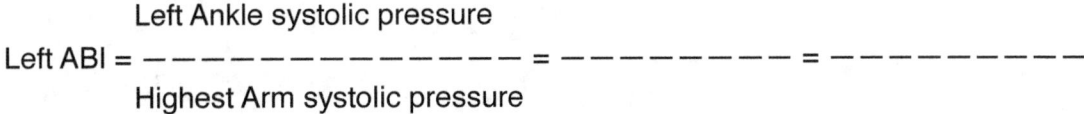

$$\text{Left ABI} = \frac{\text{Left Ankle systolic pressure}}{\text{Highest Arm systolic pressure}} = ————— = —————$$

33

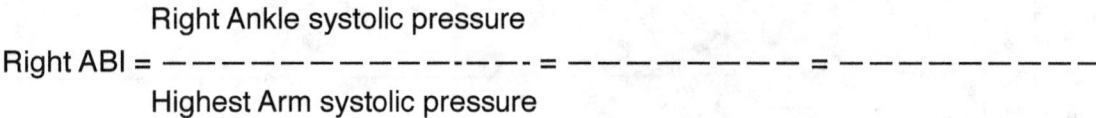

$$\text{Right ABI} = \frac{\text{Right Ankle systolic pressure}}{\text{Highest Arm systolic pressure}} = \underline{\qquad\qquad} = \underline{\qquad\qquad}$$

ABI / Severity of Disease:

\> 1.40 = Noncompressible

1.00 - 1.40 = Normal

0.91 - 0.99 = Borderline

0.00 - 0.90 = Abnormal

Creager MA, et al. (2011). 2012 ACCF/AHA/ACR/SCAI/SIR/STS/SVM/SVN

Instruments Recommended

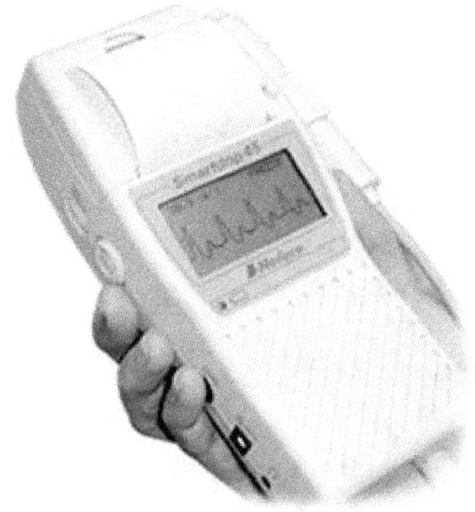

Smartdop® 45 Vascular Ultrasound Doppler

Koven Technology, Inc.
12125 Woodcrest Executive Drive, Suite 320
St. Louis, MO 63141
Michael Stahlschmidt, Sales
800-521-8342 ext. 51
$2,500

Accessories
VC-12 12 mm vascular cuff ($44)
VC-12 12 mm vascular cuff ($44)
VC-10 10mm vascular cuff ($44)
VC-10 10mm vascular cuff ($44)

Sphygmomanometer (SPG-1) ($85)

Doppler Printer Paper (PA-1) ($38)

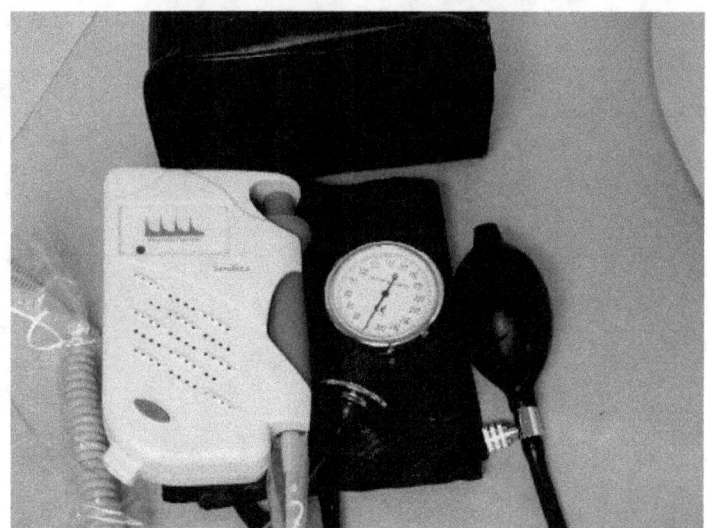

Edan Sonotrax Vascular Doppler 8 MHz probe, ABI kit (including sphygmomanometer)
East Shore Medical Supply
www.eastshoremedical.com
866-376-9944
order with 8 MHz probe and large adult cuff.
$122

This instrument does not have a printer or display and is limited to ABI pressure testing only.

Testing Equipment and Supplies

Equipment

www.steeles.com

Littman Master Classic II Stethoscope, 27", Item 2144L, $83.99

Welch Allyn Tycos Family Practice Blood Pressure Kit, Item 5098-23CB, $201.64

Braun ThermoScan Pro 4000, Ear Thermometer, Item 04000-200, $161.54

Amazon.com

Omron HBF-514C Body Composition Analyzer, $75.00

Abbott FreeStyle Lite Blood Glucose Monitoring System, $19.00

Abbott FreeStyle Lite Glucose Test Strips - 100 ct., $55.00

OneTouch Delica Lancing Device, $15.00

OneTouch Delica Lancets 100 ea, $11.00

www.koven.com

Smartdop 45 Vascular Ultrasound Doppler, $2,500.00
Cuffs (4 x $44 = $176)
Sphygmomanometer (SPG-1) ($85)
Doppler Printer Paper (PA-1) ($38)

www.eastshoremedical.com

Edan Sonotrax Vascular Doppler 8mhz probe, ABI kit, $122

www.bestmessage.com

Best Message 30" Massage Table, $100.00

Testing Supplies

www.drugstore.com

Bayer Multistix 10 SG Urine Reagent Strips, $63.49

Micro Essential Laboratory, Inc, 4224 Avenue H, Brooklyn, NY 11210 (718) 338-3618

Hydrion S/R Dispenser 4.5 - 8.5, Catalog#: 2210, $7.36
https://www.microessentiallab.com

Amazon.com

Metagenics Zinc Tally Liquid 4 oz. (for Zinc Taste Test) $18.00